FOREWORD

A compelling true story of the battle against electromagnetic radiation. During many years working on the leading edge of modern technology, Barry was unaware of the electromagnetic fields that were to have such an impact on his later years. Marlene had been unwell for some considerable time with vague M.E. type symptoms. It was only after the diagnosis of Alzheimer's that Barry took a journey back in time in order to find the cause. The results were intriguing, leaving more questions than answers.

NOWHERE TO HIDE

Early Awareness

I was only about seven years old when I became aware of the invisible invader. It couldn't be seen, smelt, tasted, heard, or even touched, but it was there alright. The bush radio was unable to rid itself of the invader's annoying interference. This high-tech. state-of-the-art, household possession took pride of place in our front room, (no-one had a lounge in those days, the room was either front or back). Anyway, it was near the window usually sat on granny's singer sewing machine. Clearly it was in the window for a reason, but at my tender age I hadn't understood that a radio needs some form of signal. When it was used in the back room, dad had to mess around with a coat hanger to make the thing work.

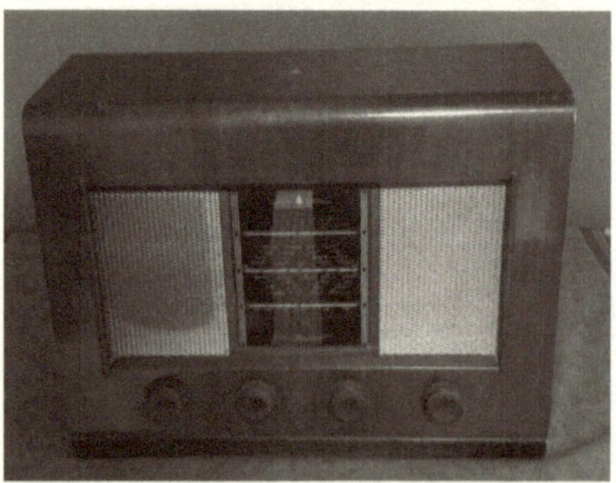

When it was working, I recall listening to most of the popular programs of the day. I was a bit old for 'Listen with mother', but I do remember 'Journey into space' and 'Flash Gordon'. It was while listening to these broadcasts that the invisible menace was unable to keep its existence a secret. Each time a car or motorcycle came up the road you could tell it was there long before you could hear the engine, it would start with an annoying click—click and grow into a steady staccato rhythm as the machine passed. Technology soon became available to suppress the interference and it became law to fit suppression devices to all vehicles. The electronic pulse was still there, just hidden. I can't imagine that in these exciting times any thought was given to any possible adverse effects on our human body. Engineers would soon find ways to improve radios and the up-coming televisions in order to include technology that would MASK the unwanted radiation that was becoming more and more prevalent in our homes.

Dad was always interested in the latest technology and as a senior foreman at the Leyland motors factory in Farrington, he was in charge of some of the most advanced equipment in the field of heat treatments. The machines used massive amounts of energy for the induction-hardening process and, as a result, a new power plant was built near the tank factory on Centurion Way. It wasn't only Leyland that needed more energy, power stations continued to be introduced to the national grid with pylons and cables crisscrossing the country like a giant spiders' webs supplying power to the ever-growing domestic market and in the process, producing more and more invisible electromagnetic fields.

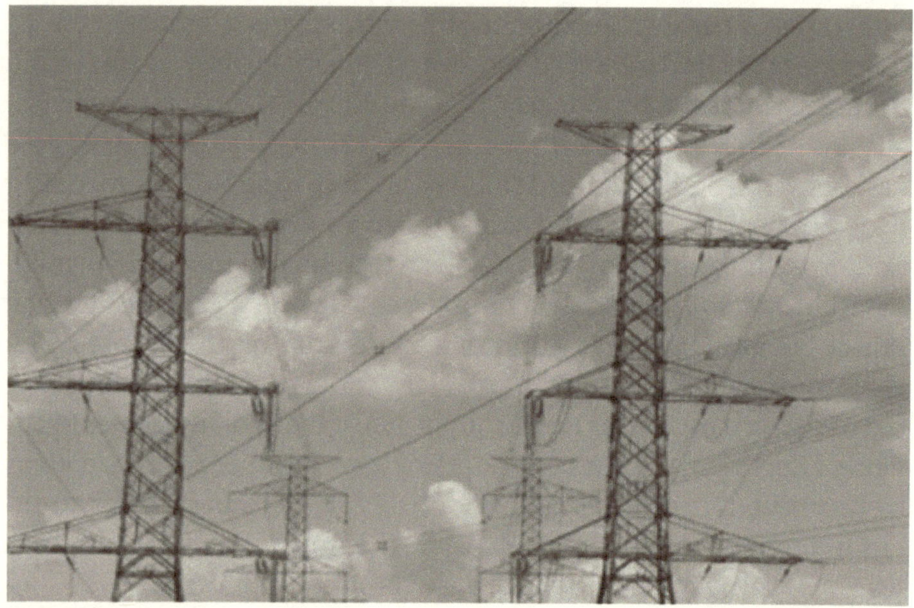

Consumer demand for TVs and all the exciting new home devices took off - vacuum cleaners, washing machines, even electric fires entered our homes. Dad managed to persuade mum that a TV was essential in order to make the most of 1953. It was to be an amazing year for the BBC; they televised the coronation and Preston North End at Wembley. A new mast had been erected on winter hill. The transmitted pulses allowed us to watch the magic of a 425-line transmission create a grainy image on screen as the set warmed up. The signal power must have been quite strong, often there was a multiple image like a ghostly shadow following every movement. Engineers spent a long time adjusting the aerials in order to minimise the effect. Signal bounce was caused by the signal reflecting from nearby buildings. I wonder if they bounced off our bodies.

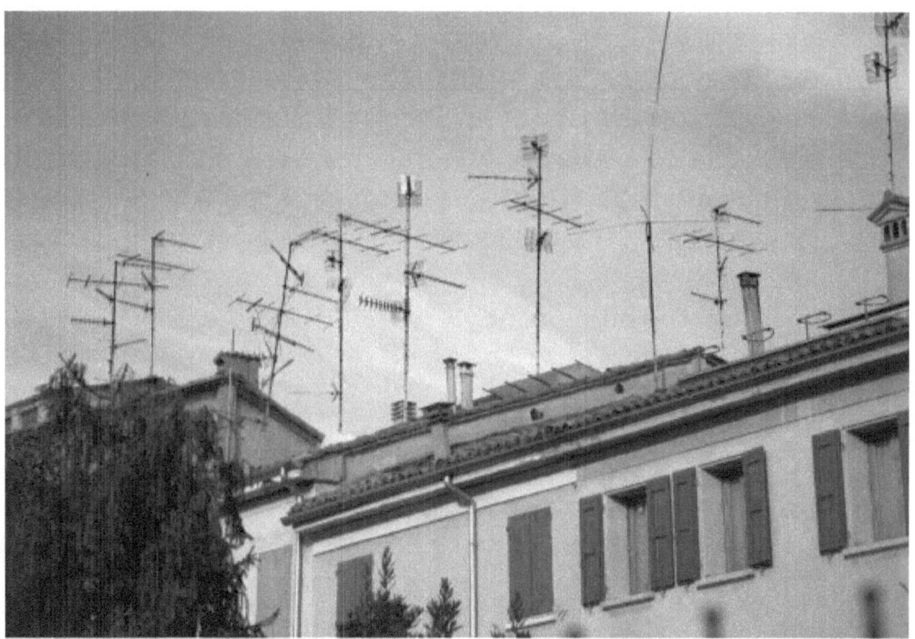

The problem was of course, that no equipment had been invented that was capable of measuring the voltage in our bodies, anyway no-one was interested; it was assumed that as long as you didn't touch the bare wires, you would be safe. I can't help but thinking of the pioneering engineers that died from shocks before the dangers became common knowledge.

Growing up as a child of the 50s was a privilege that no-one on this earth will ever experience again, with scientific breakthroughs beyond the imagination of our forefathers. There were ships, trains, planes, rockets, and nuclear power along with the conquest of mountains and the polar regions. Science-fiction was becoming a science fact, nothing would stand in the way of human endeavour, but only with hindsight would we be able to see the full picture.

Our parents must have found life hard at the time; there was still some remnants of wartime rationing and housing was still quite basic - stone floors, pot sinks, outside loos and open coal fires. We did have electric lights, but only had two electric sockets - one in each of the downstairs rooms. They were large, dark-brown boxes looking somewhat out of place on the skirting board. They were only able to power one thing at a time and, as a result, extension leads snaked their way across the room to feed other devices, whilst at the same time bombarding the unsuspecting occupants with magnetic fields that were untested in relation to their effects on the human body.

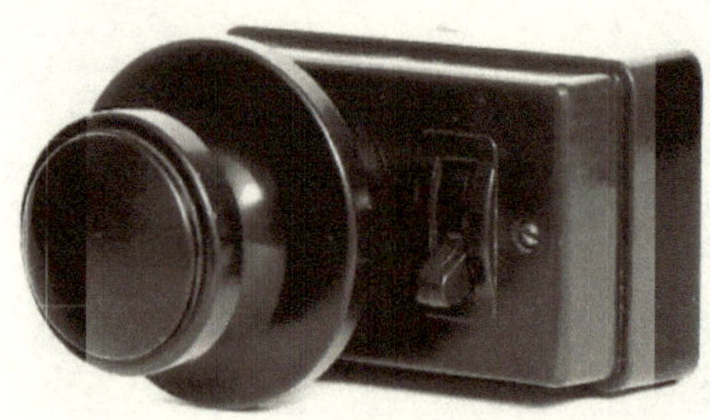

Clothing was predominantly wool, or cotton and footwear was made from organic materials such as leather or wood. (Clogs were great fun - me and my mates would see who could make the best sparks on the cobblestone path, as long as mum didn't see us). But at least we were well earthed. Yeah, we were fine, but the sinister underlying effects of technological advancement was little understood. Whilst diphtheria, TB and other common illnesses were on the decline and morality rates improved, new conditions were emerging of which we had little understanding. Energy use had been increasing significantly since the turn of the century and the first diagnoses of Alzheimer's came in 1910, along with many more neurological diseases in the pursuing years.

The graph shown below is from the office of national statistics. It is similar to many other graphs that depict the rise of many modern-day conditions and illnesses. It is not my objective to bombard the reader with selective data that would support my case. Check it out for yourself

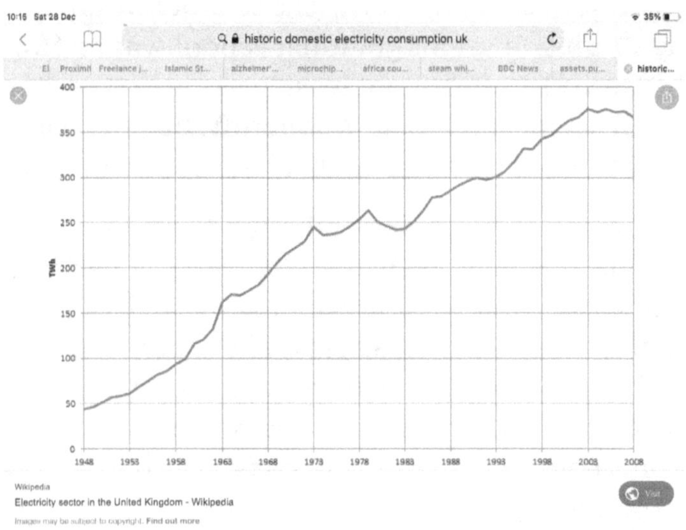

Early Youth

My childhood behind me, it was time to move on to my educational years. The family moved home in 1955 to an abandoned scrap yard on the outskirts of Longton. The price of £1,800 reflected the state of the place; scrap metals and abandoned cars littered the five-acre site, but that didn't deter my dad. It would soon become a small holding. With a bit of hard work, the sale of the scrap did, in fact, go a long way toward paying the Chorley building society. Pig pens and fencing were the first priority; the leaky roof and repairs to the bungalow would have to wait - after all, it was still fit to live in.

Mum and dad made sure that we were all well taken care of and the available rooms were cleaned made comfortable and allocated accordingly. The girls had one room and I had the other.

The back-room accommodation was for my three sisters. Carol, who was the eldest, was in her final years at Balshaws grammar school in Leyland. Norma was next eldest and attended

Worden high school; she was soon to move to the newly built Penwortham secondary modern, (the school I would attend after failing my 11 plus. It seems grammar school was not for the only boy of the family). Last, but not least, was my little sister Pauline. I don't recall seeing a pram at Woodcroft, but she was still very young. How they all managed in that back room is beyond me.

My passage through secondary school education was fairly uneventful I was not good or bad at anything in particular. I was still a bit of a loner and certainly not happy with team sports; the cross-country team was the nearest I got to group activity. It was my thirst for knowledge away from school that proved the most useful in later years. The abandoned scrap cars and discarded army surplus equipment littering the field at home proved to be the most interesting.

Again, the mystery of electricity had my attention. I had often had shocks from sparkplug leads and knew how powerful they could be. I worked out that if I could figure out a way to make a windshield wiper motor turn a distributor, by connecting the sparkplug leads to an uninsulated cable around the pig enclosure, I would have an electric fence. Bingo! I had the required electric fence (I also had several burns, along with a few sore fingers but hey, what the heck!) I was pleased with it and the pigs soon learned to keep away from my creation. Job done.

Life at Woodcroft continued at a pace - mum and dad working hard, dad on nights at the motors and mum on late shift at the Longton arms. The older girls were now young women and it was Carol's job to baby-sit the rest of us.

Carol was later married to Ronnie and moved away. Norma later married Brian and on their wedding day the back room was transformed into the honeymoon suite. Instead of trying to sabotage their sleeping arrangements, I found another way to ruin their night, it came in the form of a car battery, a car horn, a time switch and some very thin 'not fit for purpose' electric wires. The contraption was duly assembled, set to activate at 2:00 am, then hidden in a cardboard box in the wardrobe. When zero hour arrived, things didn't go exactly according to plan; the timer functioned ok and the horn blasted out enough sound to awaken the whole household, but that's when it all went horribly wrong.

The wires feeding the horn melted the insulation, setting fire to the cardboard box and filling the wardrobe with toxic fumes! Fortunately, Brian was out of bed and made it safe before anybody realised what had happened. The toxic smell of burning wire lingered for a little while and Brian didn't seem to hold it against me, so the incident was soon forgotten. For my part, the memory of the danger posed by my stupidity during that night still lingers, but on the positive side I learned more about the hidden power of electricity. Never again would I build a circuit without due consideration being given to the cable capacities and fusing arrangements.

I left school at fifteen and was destined for a Leyland Motors apprenticeship. I was still interested in all things electrical and hopefully I would be able to do the electricians course. Unfortunately, it wasn't for me; the requirements for good grades in maths and english eliminating that choice. I was, however, well pleased with an offer of a place in the engineering department as a turner.

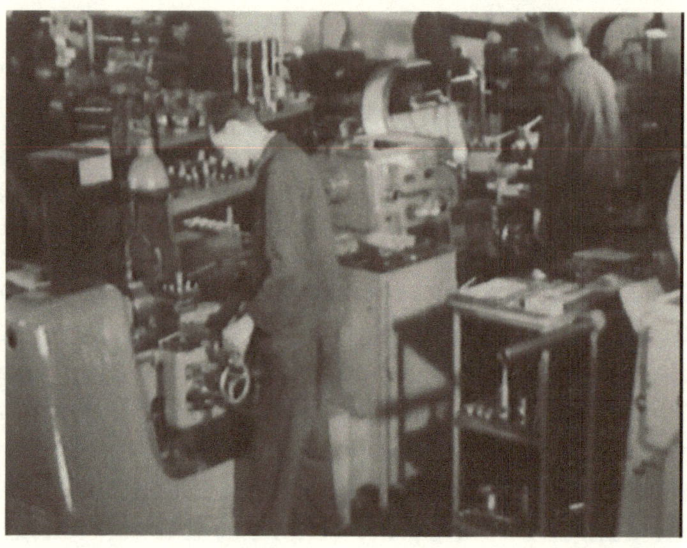

On my first day at work all the new intake were gathered together in the conference room and introduced to the apprentice superintendent, Mr Harry Glasbrook. He was a sturdy giant of a man and looked like the type of guy you wouldn't want to cross. He had all the assets of the stereotypical sergeant major with the heavy eyebrows and handle bar moustache. He was, in fact, ex-army and employed for his disciplinary skills rather than any engineering talent he may have acquired. He ruled with a rod of iron and no one broke Harry's rules, not if he was watching at any rate.

The training centre was filled with an array of lathes and milling machines of all shapes and sizes and in contrast to many of the machines in the main factory they were all independently powered, each with its own motor and control system. Over the years we had machines allocated according to our abilities. They were located in various parts of the building. It is only on reflection that I now realise that two of the machines in the corner of the workshop were rarely in use - it seems they were only allocated as a last resort, there was nothing wrong with them, but it was somehow uncomfortable working there. The main workshop carried the background noise of the machines, but in that corner was a continuous sinister background humming that made you feel really uncomfortable. It emanated from the giant bank of electrical distribution boxes on the wall. I, for one, avoided the area.

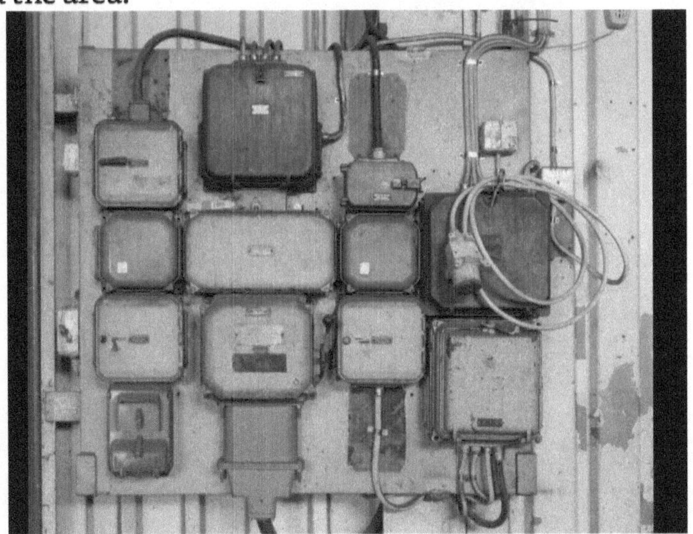

Whilst continuing with my apprenticeship, most of my spare time was spent on the scrap yard salvaging parts and selling them to colleagues at work. It wasn't long before the revenue from my little venture far exceeded my apprenticeship wages; seventeen and sixpence as I recall, handed to mum unopened, she gave me five shillings back for my dinner money. By the time I was seventeen a fully functional Morris 12 with a heater and traficators was ready for the road. There was no M O T in those days but I did have to pass my driving test.

By selling army surplus electric irons for ten shillings each and a few car parts to my workmates at Leyland Motors, I was able to escape from Longton and venture into the outside world in my new *car*. Heskin was my first adventure where I went to the local youth club with a friend from work. After that a trip to Chorley. The Tudor dance hall became a regular Saturday night adventure for me and my mate Jim. Live bands playing the latest Beatles music, gorgeous girls; well, what can I say? At seventeen years old, what's not to like?

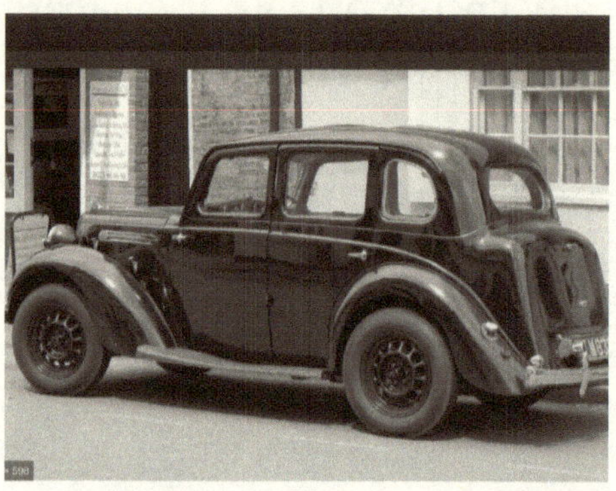

One fateful Saturday night at the Tudor was to change my life for-ever. My attention was drawn as soon as I walked in. She was tall, blonde and glided across the room with an air of confidence, with all the guys competing for some sort of eye contact with her. I knew within seconds that I wouldn't stand a chance. I would have to look elsewhere.

Boy am I glad I did! Although as beautiful as any other girl in the building in a physical sense, it wasn't the fullness of body or starched skirt that drew me to Marlene, it was something else that I still can't explain even to this day. Watching her dancing around her handbag had me totally mesmerised. Jim said, "Bet you half a crown, you don't ask her to dance." Jim lost his money and his free ride home. I didn't just win his money, I won the girl of my dreams - Marlene. I married her on 27th February 1965. The rest is another story.

Longton Motor Salvage

For the start of our married life, Marlene and I moved into an old caravan at the scrapyard. We soon made it home with hot water and a proper loo in a shed at the back. Selling scrap was to become our main source of income, so my apprenticeship was cut short in the hope that our new business would provide a better way of life. Dad was none too happy; Smiths had always been Motor's men, with steady wages and job security. He thought my plans were foolhardy and carried too much risk.

Sadly, my dad would never be able to share in our success. He arrived home from work one afternoon complaining of a headache, which was very unusual for dad, apart from the occasional cold I really don't recall seeing him poorly. After he helped me finish loading the scrap I drove off to Preston, sadly never to see him again. It was after attending the local surgery, he returned home and went straight to bed. I was told that he died within the hour. The cause of death was recorded as cerebral haemorrhage. I have no reason to doubt those finding, though as far as I can establish no one tried to find out what weakened the blood vessels in the first place.

The fact he was a healthy middle-aged male with little in the way of previous health problems, a non-smoker or drinker, should have been grounds for further investigation. That didn't happen. It would be another 40 years before compulsory safety regulations were introduced. There was obviously a need to protect people from the dangerous radiation emitting from those high-powered induction hardening machines.

I have no medical qualifications, though it would be impossible to look back at the situation today without at least considering the possibility that he got too close. If that was the case then an aneurism could easily have formed causing his headache. The doctor probably gave him a blood thinner as a precautionary measure. No one could have predicted the results.
After dad's death, Marlene and I purchased the scrapyard, Mum and Pauline moved to Croston and we vacated the caravan in favour of the bungalow.

Over the next few years we gradually grew the business. It was hard work and Marlene often helped me cutting up the cars; oxy-acetylene was uneconomical, so we resorted to using an axe to chop through the thin body material. The inevitable was bound to happen - Marlene missed her target. I thought she would bleed to death! With a car seat cover wrapped tightly around her arm, I drove her to the surgery. Dr Wilkinson did a leisurely sewing job on her while discussing the kids and the nice weather. Next thing I know I had fainted, with everyone gathered around laughing at me.

Marlene's accident spurred me on to building a car crusher, there was no way our limited income would support purchasing a new one. My new creation worked well, making the work far easier - blades moved by powerful hydraulic rams sliced into the cars and pressed them into manageable pieces that we could easily sell. Pushing the control levers back and forth all day soon became very boring. My machine needed an automated control system. That was to become quite a challenge; after all it wasn't something I could buy from Woolworths or anywhere else for that matter - a few bits from the scrap yard had proved not fit for purpose. Now was the time to venture into the world of electronics.

I found the whole thing to be really hard going. For a start my academic strengths were somewhat limited, yet here I was wishing I had paid more attention during Maths and English at school. A few surplus relays from a telephone exchange and many hours of reading books beyond my understanding, put me on the right track. It was the constant failure and trying again that finally secured the required results.

I now had a fully automated car crushing machine, I also had a heavily pregnant Marlene and a local newspaper pressing for a story about our unconventional achievements. The story ran along the lines of, "Which comes first, baby or a bale? We were famous! Lancashire evening post carried my photo beneath the headlines.

After that newspaper article a new business was born - Longton Machinery Supplies. L M S was now into manufacturing car balers at the rate of one a month and needed larger premises as a matter of urgency. After building the first industrial unit at Walton Summit, media coverage came thick and fast; a ministerial visit resulted in worldwide publicity and overseas sales.

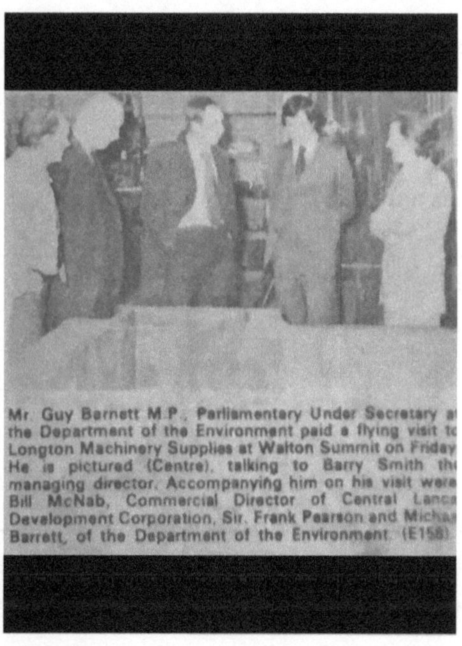

Mr. Guy Barnett M.P., Parliamentary Under Secretary at the Department of the Environment paid a flying visit to Longton Machinery Supplies at Walton Summit on Friday He is pictured (Centre), talking to Barry Smith the managing director. Accompanying him on his visit were Bill McNab, Commercial Director of Central Lancs Development Corporation, Sir. Frank Pearson and Michael Barrett, of the Department of the Environment. (E158)

It wasn't long before other companies showed an interest in L M S, and in 1976 Edbro Holdings became the new owners. Working as a non-executive director on the board of Edbro wasn't for me, it provided an income but very little else.

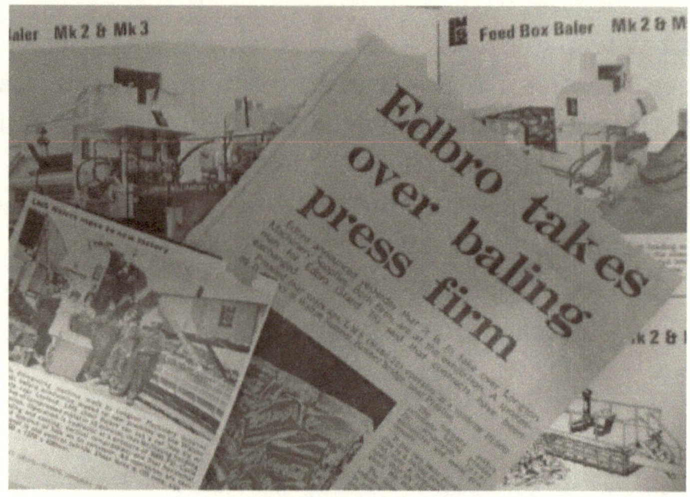

Computer sales were predicted to rise in the coming years. Not everyone agreed, although the BBC had created a surge in interest with the BBC Micro - (Amstrad and Sinclair were soon to follow). My attention was drawn to the IBM recruitment day being held at Manchester university. Armed with my CV and full of confidence, I sat in the lecture hall expecting to be called for an interview. When I was handed an exam paper my naivety suddenly dawned on me; all the other candidates knew an exam was the first stage, the last time I did any sort of exam was my eleven plus, and I failed that.

Not having been selected for interview, I took the train journey home reflecting on my stupidity. The humiliation I felt was irrational, but I vowed never to put myself in that position again. If I B M didn't want to avail themselves of my considerable talents, then I would have to start my own computer company.

At the time my daughter Nicola was learning to play the electronic organ, which involved learning chords and scales by following drawings and diagrams in a colourful little book. How much easier it would become if the finger positioning could be displayed instantly at the touch of a button. Technology for that sort of thing was in its infancy, but with help from Hitachi and permission from Sir Clive Sinclair to use his keypad manufacturing process, I had the makings of a business venture. The name 'Prelude' was derived from the musical term, meaning, '

"to precede" or "beginning." If successful we would indeed have the first hand-held electronic book. After a great deal of work the Prelude chord computer was born.

Prelude Electronics

Prelude electronics was originally formed for the sole purpose of, the manufacture and distribution of chord computers. Great TV coverage and excellent reviews in newspapers and magazines helped to ensure its success. We were soon exporting to music stores worldwide.

Prelude had become an electronics manufacturer and was to learn the pitfalls the hard way. Our failure rate was far too high and biting deeply into our profitability. In desperation, a batch of microprocessors were returned to Hitachi for failure analysis. They responded with a detailed technical report, including a recommendation to change our manufacturing process in order to reduce the risk of static damage. After introducing full static control procedures, our failure levels were reduced to almost zero. This was to be the start of my studies into this phenomenon, ultimately allowing Prelude to become a well-respected electronics company.

The huge success of the product was actually to be its downfall; the earlier failures had prevented us from achieving the rapid expansion required to take advantage of our early lead. Cassio, and later Corg, flooded the world market with similar products within a year of our first sales. Our sales didn't just slowdown; they stopped almost overnight, which left us with financial problems. My American agents still preferred Prelude so I sold him the manufacturing rights and he contracted us to manufacture them for him.

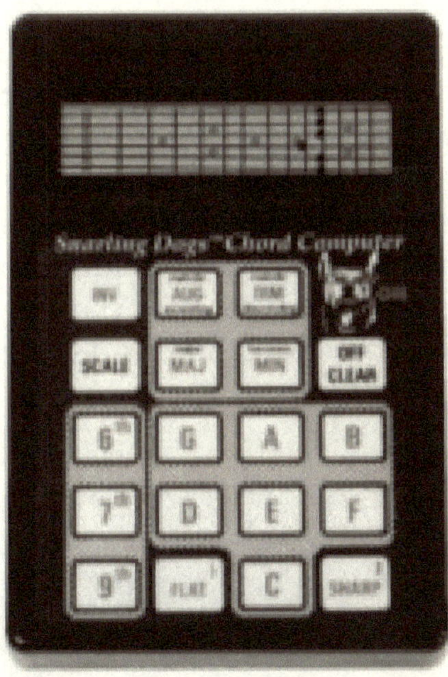

Prelude effectively became the assembly contractor, thereby en-abling supply of the chord computer to continue, (albeit under a new brand name of Snarling Dogs).

The idea of just assembling a finished product was a sound busi-ness planI didn't have the responsibility of sourcing the compo-nents and ultimately paying for them, assembly test and shipping was the main function of the business. I just had to swallow my pride as far as the chord computer was concerned. It would be some time before I had a product of my own again, in the meanwhile we manufactured a broad range of products for other companies. By minimising electromagnetic radiation within the workshop and training all the personnel to follow the static pre-caution guidelines, we were able to provide an excellent manu-facturing service, with little or no static damage to the finished product. As a responsible company, we followed all the statutory requirements of the health and safety at work act. Even then, I still thought that the only danger from electricity was electric shock.

As the business expanded our customers required a much more inclusive service involving the procurement and stockholding of the specialist components. A move from Walmer Hall to Liverpool Road enabled that expansion. What used to be a plumber's workshop was soon transformed into a modern assembly unit with all the storage and automated soldering equipment at our disposal. The first big order was from the record company EMI. Pink Floyd released a special album in 1995 called 'Pulse, Dark Side of the Moon'.

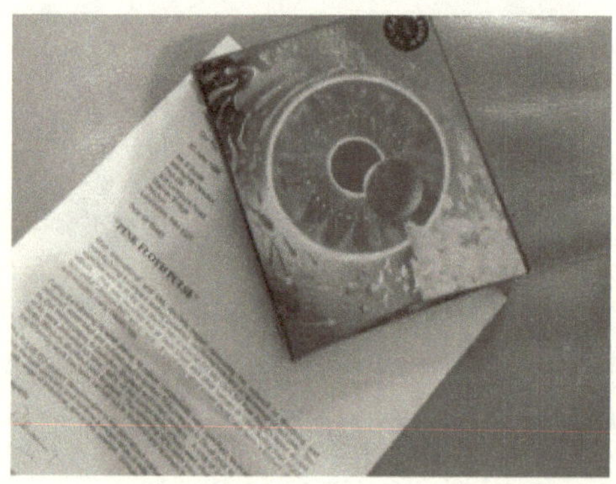

The logistics of completing this order was quite staggering. Can you imagine the weight of a box containing 20,000 AA batteries? It was a tough contract with stringent quality control, but it established Prelude as a serious player in the electronics business. We now had equipment and personnel to develop our own products, the first of these was the digital audio recording system.

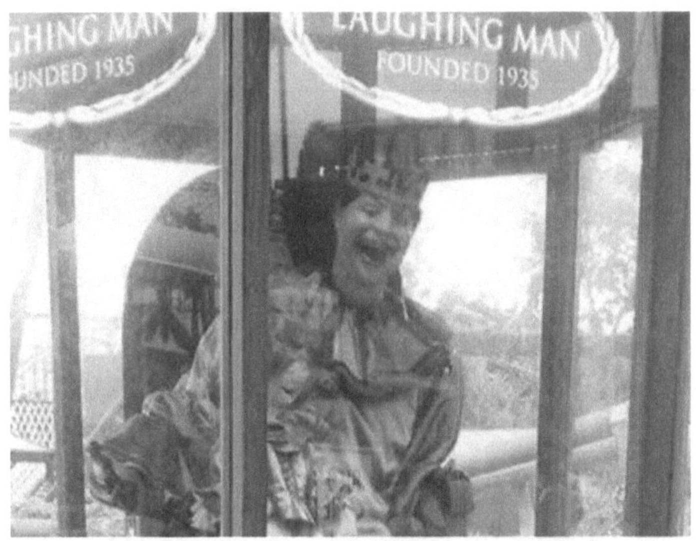

The equipment was included in the Farnell catalogue with a few encouraging sales, but the most high-profile application was the upgrading to digital audio of the laughing man at Blackpool pleasure beach. Over a period of time we converted the entire theme park.

Another addition to Prelude products was the domestic waste compactor. It fit neatly under the kitchen worktop and was easily capable of crushing a full week's worth of household waste into a neat little block. The engineering aspects of the product were fairly easy, but with the recent introduction of the CE mark, alongside all the compulsory regulation related to white goods manufacturing, the project was far from straight-forward.

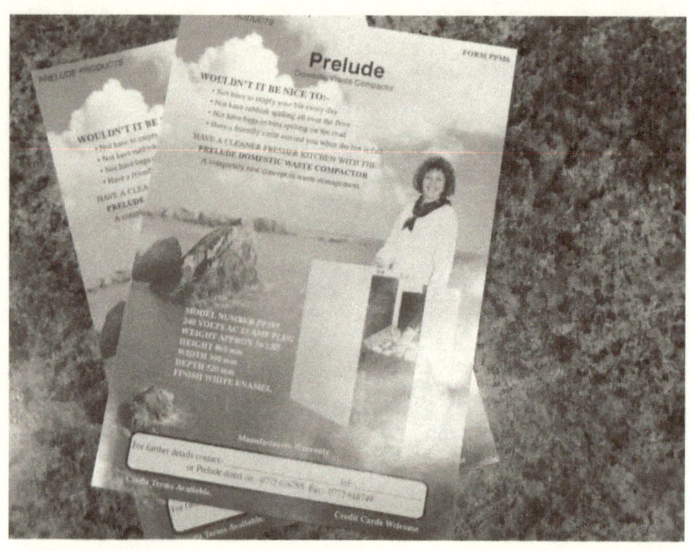

Mechanical safety concerns were soon overcome, but the electrical issues proved to be far more complex The physical aspects as regards electrical insulation, fuses and earthing was again straight-forward but yet again I came across the invisible menace.

Electromagnetic fields were supposed to be harmless, yet here we were approaching the last days of the twentieth century and what appeared to be stringent regulations controlling these invisible fields were to be legally enforced. All I was interested in was getting the necessary certification for my product. On reflection, looking at it two decades later, the regulations were not stringent enough. I recently discovered that the EMC part of the requirement was a regulation that required manufacturers to ensure emissions did not interfere with other electronic devices nearby. It was NOT to protect the health of people.

The Regulations

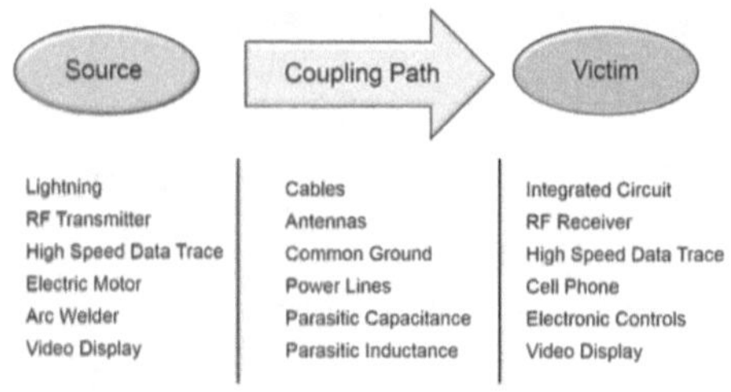

Figure 1. The three essential elements of an EMC problem.

e nuclear power plant, the receptor was readily identified. The turbine control valves were ma
known; however an investigation revealed that wireless handsets used by the plant employees
known, the problem was solved by eliminating the source (e.g. restricting the use of low-power r

It seems that the requirements were initially drafted following the loss of a Boeing 747. Air crash investigators established the cause was electrostatic discharge in the fuel tank, from a source unknown. At the time an immediate ban on the use of electronic equipment on board flights came into force.

In order to acquire the necessary CE mark certification, the test had to be carried out by an authorised contractor. It involved positioning sensors 50 cm from the compactor and recording various readings. It didn't occur to me then that' in order to use the equipment, an operator would have to be in contact with the machine, not stood away from it.

After various modifications and component changes we came very close to achieving the required standards, but not close enough. eEen outside on our car park the additional background radiation prevented the issuing of the necessary certificates. Certification was eventually issued after the tests were carried out in a controlled environment at Manchester university.

The facilities in Manchester were soon to be used again, this time to control magnetic fields in the opposite direction. Our contract with Exide was to develop and produce a security device that would disable the car unless the desired signal was received from a hand-held key fob. In those days cars still needed a key, anti-theft devices were relatively rare. The task of designing a device that was capable of reacting to a pre-selected radio signal and yet still able operate amid all the interference generated from within the car was not down to me.

The engineers used the Manchester test chamber to bombard the device with all kinds of invisible electrical radiation. Even with my close involvement in all this technology I had still never seen or even heard of anyone measuring body voltage. The equipment was common and readily available, but no one was concerned. We were becoming more and more isolated from the earth with highly insulated footwear and synthetic clothing. That was not my concern at the time, after all electromagnetic fields are not harmful. RIGHT?

My priority was to win the manufacturing contract and in order to achieve that goal, a larger factory and installation of highly sophisticated manufacturing equipment was required. The lingerie company at Walmer Bridge had recently been liquidated leaving ideal premises available only a short distance from our existing building. It was in a reasonable state of repair and importantly had good vehicle access and a power supply adequate for our needs.

With the contract secured, work started on the refurbishment of the factory and installation of various equipment and the production line. One of the requirements was that Prelude must ensure a static-free environment. This had nothing to do with the safety of our personnel, but rather the safety of the microprocessors used in the manufacturing process. Since scientists discovered that failure of many electronic components was due to discharge of electricity from the human body, it has been a requirement to keep personnel grounded by means of special footwear and wristbands. The damage to components from human contact can be extensive.

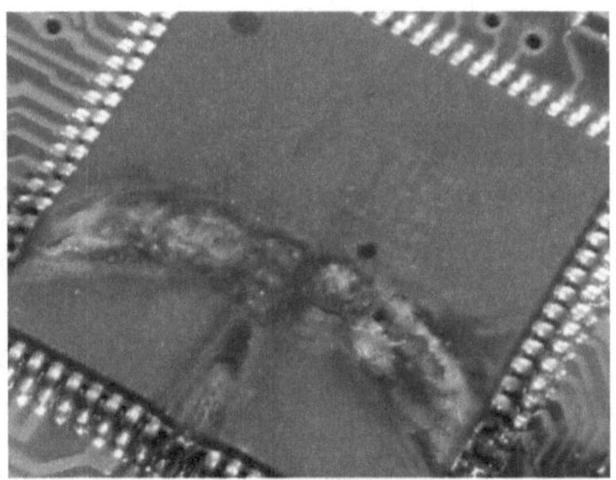

Considering those man-made microprocessors are probably thousands of times more robust than the human neurological system, is it not reasonable to assume that as electricity builds in our bodies when not grounded. The result may just have some form of influence on our own human structures?

The new factory up and running, our reputation within the manufacturing sector enabled the company to grow steadily. We made a broad range of electronic equipment for use in all sorts of consumer products - telecommunications, medical, security, the list was growing. However the additional workload was a significant challenge for me personally.

The day started early, all jobs were allocated to the available staff by the time they arrived at 8:00 am. My office was at the front of the building adjoining the electrical substation. It was comfortable, nicely furnished and well-lit. It also served as a boardroom when needed. When I started feeling unwell the most likely cause was, of course, stress. My life to that point had been far more stressful than most. I had attended high profile meetings, TV appearances, board meetings at Edbro and I had witnessed some of the worst aspects of human aggression whilst stranded at Kinshasa airport during a terrorist attack. At no time during that period did I feel so unwell.

After a while the doctors said I probably had ME. All the symptoms seemed to match, I certainly couldn't get through a full day at work. I am absolutely certain it was not ME. My office desk was placed directly against the electrical distribution boards that fed the factory. For many years I had been accused of being a workaholic and it had been suggested many times that I take up some sort of hobby away from my working environment, in order to improve my health. Being such a loner, team sports and golf were not for me. When I came across the opportunity to buy a piece of derelict land in Scorton, the idea appealed to me. It would be a place to hide and my staff would think I was playing golf. I often spent time at Scorton, up in the woods clearing out the brambles and draining the land. Although I was exerting a considerable amount of physical effort, during the following hours I felts so much better. that reinforced the theory that stress was the cause. I can look back now with a closer understanding of all the hidden forces at work and clearly put together a relationship between my working environment and my state of health. I am now convinced that my long-term close proximity to the factory's power source and the associated electromagnetic fields was detrimental to my health.

Imagine for a moment a bucket. It can be filled and emptied suddenly or poured out slowly. Your body is the same in relation to electromagnetic radiation; it fills slowly picking up energy from the cables embedded in the house walls or from TV, radio, and mobile phones. When it's full the emptying process is often physically felt as an electric shock, for example when you go to open the car door. You didn't get a shock from the car. The car got a shock from you.

Now if the bucket was full of holes, it would never get the chance to fill. Although it may be hard to visualise, we are the same. The only difference is that, in our modern world, the mechanisms by which the human body would normally discharge have become restricted or blocked. Highly insulated footwear and domestic flooring have prevented our bodies from discharging the unnatural build-up of energy to earth. That is why I felt so much better when out on the land at Scorton. Remember stone floors and clogs? You will have heard many stories of people feeling much refreshed after a holiday in the mountains or by the sea; my own GP at the time suggested a holiday may help, I'm sure that is not a coincidence. I would like to find some way of proving that stress and many associated conditions are a neurological function caused by excessive body voltage.

My time at Prelude was drawing to a close, each day was becoming harder and being in business wasn't fun anymore. The doctors couldn't find any physical reason for my illnesses so the decision to sell Prelude when the opportunity arose in 2004 was a no-brainier. My forty-three years working with and around electricity and electronic devices had been a privilege of the modern age, and at the time I was proud of my contribution to the development of many new products like digital audio systems and smart-meters. Even though over the years I had witnessed unexpected readings when test probes inadvertently touched my skin, I had still never actually measured my body voltage, and saw no reason to do so.

With the business years behind me my health gradually improved. Naturally it was assumed that the lack of stress was the reason, it would be another ten years before the original cause of that stress would become clear to me. Marlene and I spent more and more time at Scorton. It was hard work and many people openly said that the geology of the site was likely to make it beyond economic development. Plans had been approved by the local authority late in 1999. We didn't think it would take until 2008 before we moved in.

Our accommodation was at first the semi derelict bungalow. It was built close to the road and was slowly subsiding towards the river. As soon as the garage was close to completion I installed a kitchen and left a cavity beneath the car park in order to accommodate the bathroom. Before moving in, a camera was installed in order to keep an eye out for any uninvited council officials.

With the garage made habitable it was time to start on the main project, we moved in and sold the house in Longton. That enabled us to purchase the necessary building materials and equipment. With the old building demolished and major excavation work underway we began to realise the enormity of the task ahead of us but that's another story.

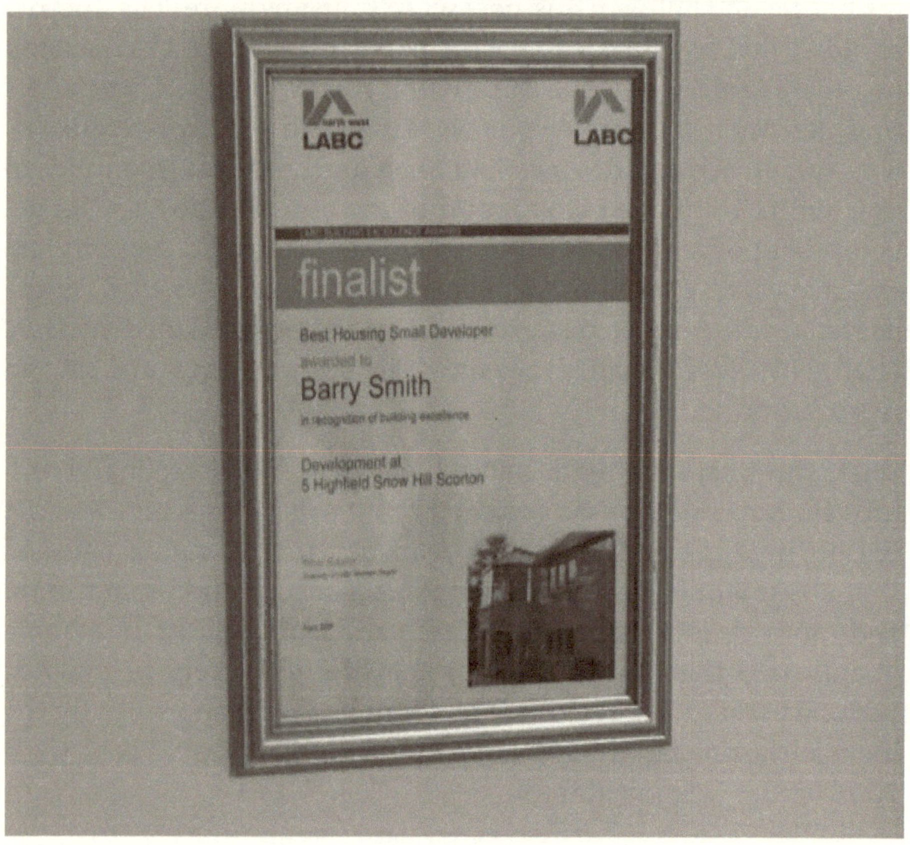

It was during the installation of tons and tons of steel reinforce-ment that a serious error was made, the consequences of which only came to light in 2016. All building control requirements had been met, in many aspects surpassed. I was even awarded the 2009 LABC building excellence award.

The error was in fact nothing I had actually done wrong, it was probably more due to the fact that the insulation and water-proofing were beyond statutory requirements. Over time, as the construction dried out, the steel bars embedded deep in the concrete became antennas, they were also surrounded by large quantities of polystyrene insulation. I had in inadvertently created a giant capacitor.

We moved into our new home in august 2008 and by Christmas we were able to host the best Christmas Day ever.

Castle Scorton

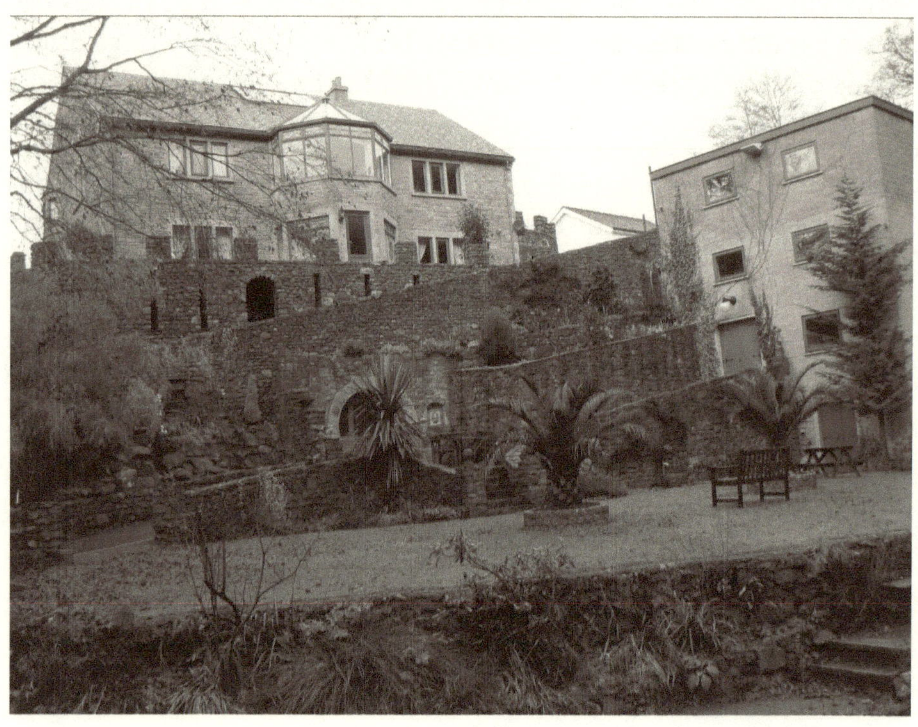

Castle Scorton, as one of my builder friends had called it, was large enough to accommodate our entire family. Marlene and I along with our three children and seven grandchildren had a Christmas that I, for one, will never forget.

The following years saw the property almost always fully occupied, at first by Nikki, Ian and the two girls. They had just purchased a bungalow down the road, it was in a beautiful location although it would require a full rebuild. That would turn out to be a substantial undertaking to which we all rose to the challenge. Ian had recently been diagnosed with breast cancer and was undergoing treatment. As a school headmaster, he had been in possession of a mobile phone for longer than most. He kept it in his breast pocket and has maintained ever since that in doing so was probably the cause of his illness. A new mobile in those days didn't come with the warning not to hold it against your body. Please don't keep your phone in your pocket or down your bra. Better still please don't keep your phone.

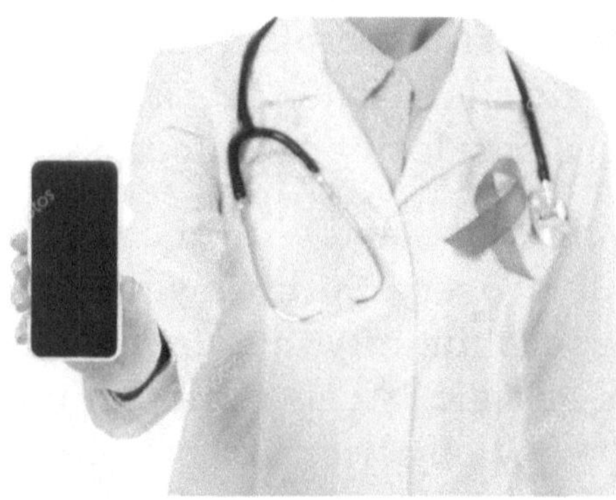

With the Cookson family ready to move on, our son Stephen brought his family from Ireland. They took residence on the top floor, sharing the kitchen with Marlene and I on the main floor. They had recently purchased the derelict Woodacre Hall located a couple of miles away. It was to be some time before that building was ready for occupation. Fortunately, the Cooksons moved on and the overlap only lasted a few weeks. Stephen's family took the upper floors, while Marlene and I made a comfortable home in the accommodation built partially below ground level.

That was early in 2011 and although very comfortable we were unaware of a well-hidden accumulation of circumstances that would eventually change our lives. The high concentration of steel used in the construction, the extensive use of thermoplastics and polystyrene for insulation, the non-conductive ceramic floors, but worst of all was the positioning of our bed. We were sleeping against a wall that turned out to be emitting electromagnetic radiation beyond WHO recommend limits. The only thing missing at that time from the equation was, in fact, time,.

It was to be another five years before the long-term cumulative effects of that exposure became clear.

We moved on to the renovation of Woodacre Hall, and spent most of our time there. On the 4th of December 2012 whilst working alone in the highest part of the building, some timbers gave way resulting in a fall through two floors. My phone was in the van parked at the front. Even to this day I find it hard believe that even with all those broken bones and an injured spine, I managed to navigate all the fallen debris, two flights of stairs and make the 999 call before losing consciousness.

I was home for Christmas and with the help of the NHS, eventually made a full recovery. During my final check-up by my GP he noticed some involuntarily muscle movements on the back of both my legs, he said it was rather an unusual occurrence and would I have any objections to him discussing it with his colleagues. I agreed and a few days later he phoned me suggesting a referral to a neurologist at the Preston hospital. Several tests were carried out and confirmed that I was suffering from peripheral neuropathy, a neurological disorder involving the neurones in the bodies electrical system not doing what they were supposed to do. Cause unknown. I had previously been diagnosed with SVT, which is another electrical problem that causes the heart to race out of control. After several 999 events they fixed that for me at Blackpool with a keyhole heart procedure called an ablation. It would seem my plumbing was good, but my wiring was shot to pieces.

Fully recovered and Woodacre Hall finally finished, Stephen and Audrey, along with their sons Andrew and Jack, moved out and our daughter and husband, Lorraine and Alastair moved in. They were missionaries working in Africa most of the time and for a while only spent short periods with us. They only moved in permanently after their work in Africa was completed.

2015 was upon us and we were about to witness a change in

Marlene's health. iI was subtle at first with symptoms much the same as when the doctors suspected I had ME, she was lethargic, depressed, and somehow not her usual self. On one occasion the pain in the muscles of her right arm almost brought her to tears so we visited our GP. After a thorough examination, blood and urine samples taken, he assured us that he would sort it out. The next day he called and told me that, although all the results were not back, the ones he had expected to be positive were not and could we return to the surgery to discuss the problem further. Marlene had always been in good health, as a non-smoker and only a light social drinker, her symptoms were somewhat vague. After arriving at the surgery, we spent some time discussing lifestyle and diet. He was obviously concerned and arranged for a colleague to perform an ECG during her lunch hour. Within minutes of the test an ambulance was called, and Marlene rushed to Lancaster hospital for further examination.

The initial response by the cardiologist's team was excellent with full emergency protocols applied. After blood tests and a further ECG, they were soon able to establish that the earlier inconclusive results were in fact a harmless irregularity unique to Marlene. She was in no immediate danger, the later referral to a cardiac consultant resulted in many trips to various hospital departments for a range of tests.

The first, as I recall was a scan involving the injection of radioactive dye. She became so stressed that it had to be abandoned. Over the following weeks her condition deteriorated - trips to the shop became a major undertaking and it appeared that any exposure to artificial environments left her feeling totally exhausted. Echocardiogram, MRI scan ultrasound, and even an unpleasant angiogram failed to provide a diagnosis. The final test was a brain scan carried out at the Kendal hospital. The consultant said images would suggest some form of physical brain injury. He repeatedly asked if she had experienced previous head trauma such as a car crash or head-surgery. I still made no connection to what I now believe to be the actual cause. After final consultations and all the tests had been analysed, the cardiologist discharged her back into the care of our local GP. The report clearly stated that apart from an abnormal ECG and slightly raised cholesterol level's, Marlene was fine. The only recommendation for treatments were the re-prescribing of a different anti-depressant and the introduction of a statin. I felt that we were no nearer, if anything her condition was getting worse.

In desperation I took to the internet. I was outside my comfort zone, desperately searching for something that would make sense. I first looked at all the medical stuff on NHS websites, most of it was too technical for me and was way over my head. Then, being drawn into some of the more obscure theories, I discovered many people have claimed that hugging trees or walking barefoot somehow had hidden powers. Marlene had always claimed that when digging in the garden she did feel better, so it would be well worth doing a bit myself and I started digging deeper. The area of alternative therapies and health improvement strategies, when seen via the internet, is a minefield to be navigated with extreme caution - theories ranging from the bizarre to the downright impossible litter search engine results.

Some cultural claims, however, did prove interesting. In particular, claims regarding Geopathic stress, not in the sense that I accepted the theory, but it did seem worthy of further investigation.

After downloading an application that was claimed to detect earth's magnetic anomalies, I gingerly moved around our home, looking for a movement on the image of a meter displayed on my iPad screen. As a non-believer, I was intrigued by the readings; as I moved around the various rooms I found a surprising variation in the radiation levels. For the most part, readings showed normal background radiation. Then, unexpectedly an alarm sounded. I retraced my steps and established that the highest readings were to be found at the bottom of the bed, on what was Marlene's side As I moved cautiously toward the bed head audible warnings reached their peak, with the corresponding gauge against its limits by the time I reached the wall. My concerns were growing.

Not yet convinced, google was tasked with the job of finding a way to disprove my findings. I wasn't prepared to spend a fortune on the equipment recommended. I found some suggestions that a magnetic compass was capable of detecting electromagnetic fields, so I ran to my workshop to retrieve a compass that was purchased when setting up my satellite dish. I knew exactly where it was, and I couldn't wait to disprove the results obtained by my free downloaded app. Unfortunately, that wasn't to be the case - it only added to the mystery. Each time I approached the bedroom wall, an error of about forty degrees registered on the dial. The compass did NOT register magnetic north.

Meanwhile Marlene's condition was not improving; she was at her worst when cooking and ironing and her best when outside in the garden. I took over the cooking and bought a drier, in the hope that she wouldn't need to iron as much. During my continuing search for answers I came across the phrase, "electromagnetic hypersensitivity". Bingo! Had I finally found the cause of Marlene's problems? The task of explaining "electromagnetic hypersensitivity" (or EHS as it is known) would be a massive undertaking. The charity ES-UK was formed to support people who are electro-sensitive They provide links to many publications and in particular a BBC interview on YouTube that will explain better than I. https://youtu.be/B73RhiP3yDc.

The theory is that, after long term exposure to a source of electromagnetic radiation, a person becomes sensitised or allergic and will often demonstrate symptoms similar to Marlene's. As an engineer I can visualise it like a fuse in an electric circuit - if you were to continually overload the fuse eventually it will blow. Recent trials that involve implanting tiny electrodes in the brain, then stimulating them using a pacemaker-like device has shown to have some remarkable results. To my mind that appears to be like replacing the fuse.

Many world governments acknowledge EHS as a medical condition. But unfortunately the official NHS recommendations for doctors presented with a patient claiming to be suffering from EHS, is to treat them for depression and if necessary, prescribe anti-psychotic drugs.

You will have heard the statement, "There is no credible evidence that the use of mobile phones is a risk to health." What about this one? "There is no credible evidence that eating nuts is a risk to health." (Unless you are allergic). It's the allergic bit that makes the difference. After gleaning as much information as possible from the charity ES-UK, I decided to purchase the equipment needed to properly survey our home. Now,with an open mind, the results confirmed my previous findings. The highest concentration appeared to be against the wall where Marlene's pillow was placed and had been for at least the last five years. From a doctor's point of view, sleeping arrangements had no bearing on a medical assessment, so I didn't even mention it in discussions with our doctor during the next visit. However, she became so distressed our doctor refered her to the mental health clinic in Lancaster.

Whilst waiting for the appointment I set about rearranging our home. The new equipment enabled me to locate various "hot spots" and adapt our daily lives accordingly. The results were staggering, I found it hard to believe that simply moving a bed would make so much difference. Armed with new test equipment we explored further afield. Visits to the local supermarkets confirmed the presence of electromagnetic radiation far above WHO recommendations, particularly in areas with freezers and display lighting. The worst areas in all cases were close to the security scanners near the exit. Over the next few weeks, I carried the equipment with me. I won't bore you with the results, but to summarise; All artificial environments, including many homes are full of electromagnetic radiation, there is "NOWHERE TO HIDE." I now only use the equipment occasionally.

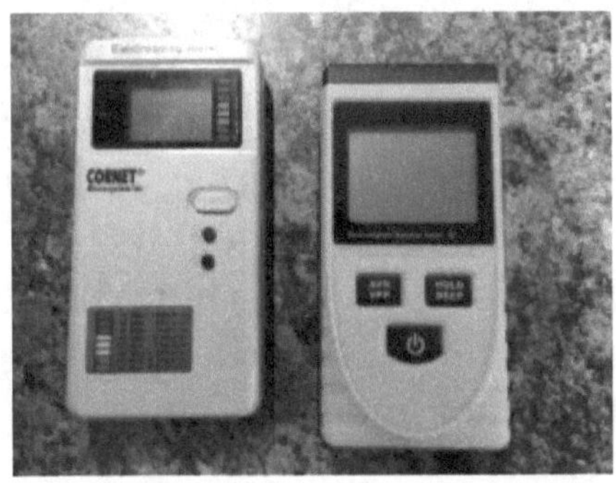

Marlene's appointment at the mental health clinic was imminent, so I wrote to the consultant in advance with the intention of making him aware of her previous exposure. During the subsequent consultation, he assured me that it had no relevance to the current investigations. After many appointments and assessments by various consultants, Marlene was eventually presented with the most cruel diagnosis of all: Alzheimer's.

Limiting Marlene's proximity to known sources of radiation had a massive positive effect on her wellbeing. We were able to establish that nausea, fatigue, headaches and general ill-health were directly related to her physical location during the preceding hours. For example, a visit to a shop or hospital would trigger the symptoms a little while later. The short-term memory was a different thing which caused frustration and anger but, apart from depression it in itself, it didn't actually make her ill.

During the next couple of years, I dedicated myself to locating and if possible eliminating sources of radiation in the home. The worst was the emission from the bedroom wall. I suspected that the embedded reinforcement may provide a clue. The prospect of having to demolish the wall receded, when I realised that I may be able to access the reinforcement from the storeroom directly below. Carrying out further tests I obtained the same results from against the store room wall as I had on the one above. After two hours with a hammer and chisel, my fingers were bleeding and bruised, another hour and I finally exposed a portion of the steel bar embedded in the wall. With blood still dripping from my fingers I struggled to connect an electrode in order to test its electrical characteristics. There was a reading of nine volts on my digital multimeter and I found that by connecting the bar to Earth, the radiation was neutralised. I felt that I was somehow taking back control by earthing anything that exhibited the ability to create a magnetic field. The kitchen proved to be the most difficult. Even the tap measured nine volts.

Two years were spent trying to shield Marlene. Each time she appeared unwell I had to work out where she had been. Then one day I realised that it wasn't just location, activity was to play a part in the equation. Ironing was put on my list of triggers. Why wasn't that spotted earlier? I purchased and installed special shielding cables but unfortunately we didn't see any significant improvements. Marlene's situation was bad enough, her independence was slowly being stolen from her. Not being able to drive any more was upsetting, now she was unable to browse her favourite shops, eat out in previously favourite places, or simply go to a supermarket. To ask her to stop ironing was not an option.

I was conscious of my own emotional decline, fully aware of the fact that no amount of feel-good pills would change the situation. My triple bypass operation in June had been a great success, allowing me to become more physically active, I was even able to replace the gutters on the house. But with winter upon us, outside activities became limited. Most of my time was spent further experimenting with ways of shielding electromagnetic radiation. The established method is to create a faraday cage around the subject. Specialist companies from around the world sell clothing and devices that are claimed to simulate that effect. I was, and still remain very sceptical. A faraday cage relies on a conductive substance surrounding the subject being connected to the earth or grounded. Much of the equipment on offer didn't fit that criteria. Earthing was of interest to me because my work in the electronics industry had left me in no doubt about the damage that static discharge was capable of inflicting on physical components.

That led me to look into claims relating to health and grounding. A whole culture and belief system has evolved in relation to reconnecting with nature. After many hours of trawling through websites and articles I became convinced that the believers can't all be nut jobs. My problem was the common denominator running through most of the articles. The phrase, "earth's natural energy." As an engineer the idea that a magical force could somehow enter their bodies through grounding didn't ring true; it was preventing me from seeing the full picture. Then it dawned on me; Mother Earth was NOT feeding them its life-giving powers. It was removing toxic electricity FROM their bodies that they didn't even know they had.

Body Voltage

For the first time since starting my research, I had a sense that I was somehow close to finding the solution. For months I had been measuring the voltage of items around the house, it hadn't occurred to me that our bodies are conductive. For the first time I used the multimeter to see if I was positively charged. There was a reading, but it didn't seem to make any sense. It was only when I adjusted the meter to AC that I realised that we are constantly bombarded with AC radiation; the national grid resonates at 50Hz. It now made sense; our bodies are conductive and as such will react to electronic signals much like a radio antenna. Whenever ever our bodies are isolated from the earth, the radiation charges us much like a capacitor.

Armed with this new information, Marlene's body voltage was

checked and was found to be 4.8v. Although we were in the same place, using the same equipment, her reading was way higher than mine. My body mass was much greater than her's, yet my reading was 1.24v. I was intrigued with these results. Could this be further proof that Marlene was indeed E H S?

Returning to the internet I found many details of research into the condition, but if my suspicions were correct I would first have to ensure that Marlene was protected as much as possible. Having now accepted that there was indeed "nowhere to hide." My searches turned to finding ways of minimising the damage caused, rather than trying to stop the unstoppable. I imagined myself in a situation where I was gradually being overloaded with work; I would pass it on, to the waste-bin or let someone else handle it. Either way, as a form of self-preservation, it would be discarded. Imagine, if you were out in a storm with no protection, unable to control the rain, with the rising water levels becoming a threat to your life.   "DRAIN THE WATER."

That would now be my goal. I must now find a way of preventing the voltage levels in Marlene from reaching a point that made her feel unwell. Surprisingly it turned out to be a relatively easy task. I ordered conductive bed sheets and pillow cases, along with a customised anti-static wrist band, (a standard wrist-band that would normally be used in the electronics industry would need the internal resistance changing to 1k). Whilst waiting for them to be delivered, I kept a close eye on the A C voltage recorded on Marlene's right hand, it was always about 50% higher than mine. There were obvious signs of negative mood changes corresponding to anything above 3.8v.

At one time she was feeling really ill with headaches and exhaustion, I hurriedly took a reading and found it to be 9.6v. She rested for a while, giving me the opportunity to check her previous actions. I found that I no longer needed the specialist radiation meter, the offender could be found by simply measuring my own body voltage as I approached the source. I could even locate hidden cables by simply moving my hand over the wall. On this occasion ironing had been the source of the problem. Continuing to explore the related science, led me to look at research in relation to the effects of electricity on the human brain. After all, the very reason for this project was Marlene's diagnosis, I needed to learn as much as possible.

Much of the information presented to me was related to the controversial treatment of psychiatric patients, but I did find useful information in relation to how the brain functions. It is actually a superior piece of electronic equipment, but unlike microprocessors that have been developed and evolved over the years, the brain functions by using electronic pulses of such a tiny magnitude that the ability to detect and measure them is a relatively modern technology. I did however learn a few interesting facts, the most important being the actual voltage at which the brain and neurological system works. It is actually only 0.00003 volts and resonates at 62 Hz. Mains electricity resonates at 50 Hz. The body's mechanisms that enable it to insulate these vital neurological circuits from outside interference must be incredibly robust. Many times in my working life I have been challenged with the effects of outside electrical interference, preventing electronic equipment from working properly and, in some cases, destroying it completely. Wouldn't it be possible for an outside influence to interfere with the correct functioning of the brain?

Increase in Variance

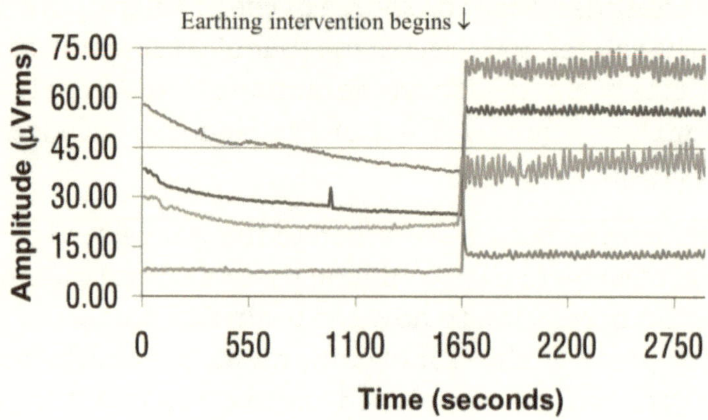

In one study, subjects were subjected to a standard EEG test in a controlled environment. Electrode pads were attached to their feet and connected to an earthing point via a switch. Constant recordings were taken for about fifteen minutes, after which time the electrodes on the feet were made active by closing the switch. Note how the strength of the signal is improved within milliseconds of earthing. I don't have a clue what this actually means but, assuming that this was a verified legitimate experiment, I am in no doubt that earthing has a direct effect on brain function.

The new wristband and bedding arrived, allowing us to start our latest experiment. At that stage I was unable to accept that something so simple could make a difference. Though I have to admit that even after the first night there was a difference. We had both slept well, which always makes us feel better anyway. Being conscious that it just may have been a psychological effect, we decided to leave our evaluation for a few days and then see how felt about it then. A few days was not required, by the following morning we were both convinced, of what exactly I don't know. Things somehow seemed more relaxed, maybe not having been disturbed with leg cramps during the night may have helped, after all it wasn't every night that it had caused a problem. Our spirits were lifted and my cramps have not returned. Only this morning Marlene checked the muscles on the back of my legs for signs of twitching, which is caused by peripheral neuropathy. Normally they are pretty obvious but this morning she had to look hard to see them.

The wristband proved to be a great asset, it achieved a reduction in voltage to less than one volt. Ironing with the wristband proved to be very effective, I had turned Marlene into a faraday cage. Power will always find the most direct route to earth, lightning for instance is the best example. A lightning conductor will protect a building from damage or fire, directing the current flow directly into the earth. Although a lot less dramatic, Marlene's wristband performs exactly the same function, leaving her unharmed. Electricity will always flow on the outer skin of the conductor, always seeking the opposite polarity, in most cases this is earth.

Day by day things were definitely improving, she was able to do household chores and rest while wearing the wristband. One Saturday a few of the family turned up all wanting a bacon butty. The cooker was on full and because Marlene had been so much better, I didn't give it a second thought. It was only after they had all gone home that she became really confused and lethargic. The muscle in her right arm was aching, and her body voltage was 9.84v. Whilst she was resting I checked where she had been cooking. We had known for years that cooking affected her and it was now routinely my job, but today I had just slipped back into our old routine. Because she had not been doing the cooking for a while, I had not checked the area. When I did I was horrified at what I found. My radiation detector had previously shown that the space around the microwave and induction hob was as to be expected an area to be avoided. This time using the multimeter my body voltage rose significantly as I approached. When touching the pan, I actually thought the equipment was faulty. After confirming the meter was ok, I took a spoon and stirred the water

- 30v, I later used an oscilloscope, with the test probe in the simmering liquid - the readings were actually, 29.84v @ 50 Hz. Although reluctant to use Marlene, on this occasion there was no other way. If my theory was correct she would be far more sensitive. Whilst stirring simmering liquid - the multimeter readings rose to above 40v in less time than it took me to switch the

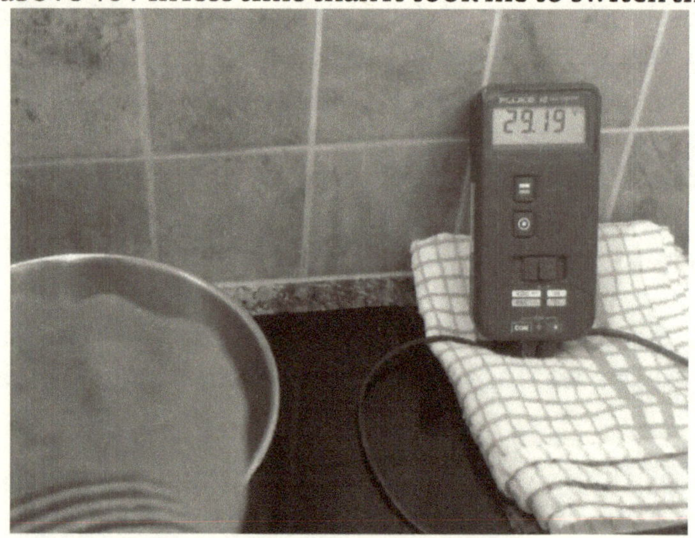

thing off. Yet more evidence that somehow Marlene's reaction to electricity was abnormal.

The induction cooker had to be replaced as soon as possible. The following day I went in search of a new gas hob unit. The first stop was my local builder's merchants, where they often had ex display and sale items. Not having a gas unit, the sales assistant suggested I install an induction hob. After explaining the reason for changing to gas, she told me that they had recently had instructions from the manufacturer not to sell induction hobs to vulnerable people with medical implants, such as pacemakers.

Finding the induction hob problem prompted me to reflect on the past few years and where all this started. Marlene's first visit to our GP was as a result of her low mood and in particular the muscle pain in her right arm. Earlier I described all the doctor's tests and results. We are now faced with the possibility that after becoming sensitised to electromagnetic radiation. The years of cooking and ironing with her right arm. Could have affected her muscle and maybe even the ECG results were somehow influenced by her illness.

Our next challenge was to find a way to keep Marlene earthed, without the restrictions of the wristband, (or dog-lead as she called it.) Lorraine and Alastair had moved into their new home in Morecambe. And it was during a recent visit that Marlene and Lorraine had occasion to visit the local supermarket. Again the symptoms returned. t was several hours before she recovered. The solution was to replace her footwear with industry standard ESD safety wear. Apart from the obvious issues relating to high heels and inadequate foot protection, the idea that the choice of footwear could affect one's health had never occurred to me. I found a few specialist suppliers catering for this market and was intrigued to find that among the main users are the NHS. Not for protecting the wearer, but to protect equipment from the wearer. I found that another major product promoted by some of these companies was ESD flooring. And among many of the users of that product are supermarkets, again not for the benefit of customers and staff but to create a cleaner environment and protect equipment from static damage.

Wearing her new ESD trainers along with conductive insoles and socks, Marlene and I cautiously ventured into our local supermarket. Being unsure of the floor's construction we didn't stay long. Whilst returning home she said she was feeling fine. Sure enough, on checking when we arrived home her body voltage was minimal. Unfortunately, within our home, the extensive ceramic flooring prevented the footwear from doing its job, so the wristband still had to be used. Further visits to that store have proved uneventful. Is it possible that at last we have a means of taking back some level of control?

I am not in denial - Marlene's diagnosis is real enough, with all the emotional problems that go with it. However, it does not seem to match the progression described in guidelines published by the Alzheimer's society. The main aspect of this is her awareness of her condition,. We have reached a point that affords us some level of hope, whether false hope remains to be seen. By keeping a close eye on the environment, we have been able to get our lives more or less back to normal. Yes, there are the short-term memory problems. Though we are now able to go shopping, do some cooking, ironing and even watching TV in the evenings without the apparent confusion experienced previously.

Only time will tell. I would love to see further research into the subject, it would be relatively easy for voltage readings to be taken during doctors' appointments. The equipment is inexpensive and easily obtainable. I don't know what the results will show, but after the last couple of years of research I have a pretty good idea. Marlene's ECG results may well have been different had she been earthed.

The Final Word

In conclusion, I must reiterate that I have no academic qualifications or medical training. I have deliberately avoided referring to specific references and research. I do not dispute the doctor's findings in any way, the support they have afforded us has been second to none. I do remain convinced, however, that the cause of Marlene's Alzheimer's is a "blown fuse" caused by 50Hz radiation. I don't personally believe that EMFs cause the actual illnesses, rather they prevent our imune system from keeping them at bay. I intend to keep Marlene "earthed" in the belief that there is a chance, with our faith and by protecting her from further damage, the miracle that is the human body will heal itself.

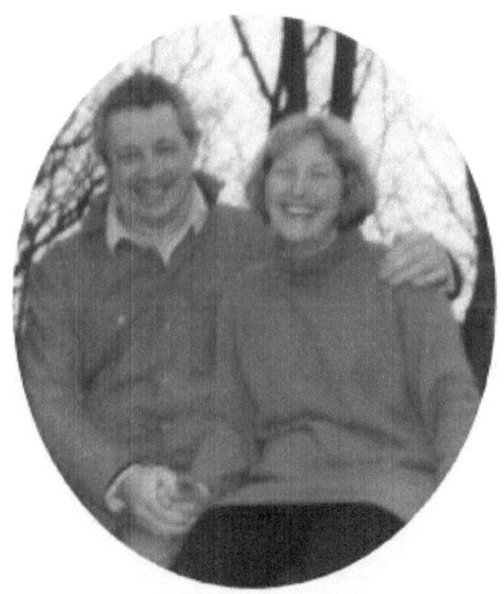

EPILOGUE

March 2020

Marlene is doing really well now with ES symptoms almost non-existent. We even spent over an hour in Asda with no ill-effects. Our goal is to promote our theories in the hope it will help others.

Thanks to

ES-UK

And of course, Marlene. My Gini pig with a doggy lead.

www.ingramcontent.com/pod-product-compliance
Lightning Source LLC
Chambersburg PA
CBHW051127250726

48655CB00007B/2935